Healthy Breasts

Every Woman's Birthright!

Healthy Breasts

Every Woman's Birthright!

Iris Ann Michael

Instant Improvement, Inc.

PURPOSE

This book is written to assist those women who would like to have more knowledge about their own Body-Temple in order to be more responsible for their health.

It is written with the hope that the health knowledge offered will become incorporated into a new lifestyle for women now as well as influence the health of future generations of women.

The information in this book is specifically directed to the subject of breast health; however, the health education presented will positively affect the health of the whole body.

I have taught professional nursing students at the diploma Associate Degree in Nursing, and at the Bachelor of Science Nursing levels. I have served as clinical mentor for Master of Science in Nursing students. At the Health Awareness Institute, I taught classes to MD's, physical therapists, psychologists, teachers, nurses, and other professionals.

With 120 women passing on with cancer EACH DAY, 44,000 needless lives lost to cancer each year, I feel this is truly a national crisis. It is not only of concern to women; it is touching every family in America.

Women throughout America are demanding preventive breast health information, but they believe there is none available. Regrettably, their attitude has been, "If my mammogram is negative, I'm fine!" That is the time to Thank God and KEEP IT NEGATIVE, instead of relaxing in a false security.

After dealing with this and other health issues for all my adult life, I feel that only now can meaningful assistance be given to you, and I am so grateful.

Iris Ann Michael

DEDICATION

To my precious daughter Pam who had the opportunity to take responsibility for her health status, to actively participate in keeping her breast clear of congestion and to take control of the process of a healthy lifestyle.

To my darling granddaughters, Katelyn Elizabeth and Savannah Mae. It is my heart's desire that you will use the Laws of health as the basis for your lifestyle and experience the wholeness of which we are all intended to participate in, experience, and enjoy.

ACKNOWLEDGEMENT

My gratitude to my children Pam, Mark, and Greg, for their faith in me and for their support and encouragement. To Dan Humphrey for computer expertise, to Nada Hornback for encouragement and editing, and to Anne Grant for her final editing of the manuscript.

DISCLAIMER

Education is freedom. The purpose of this book is for health education. None of the information in the book is to be used for, or interpreted as diagnosing, prescribing or treating any condition or disease.

Any woman finding a "lump" in her breast should see her physician immediately.

Detailed anatomy and physiology have been omitted. Graphic descriptions have been included to further the understanding of the reader concerning the design and function of their Body-Temple.

"Knowledge is your key to good health."

Benjamin Franklin

CONTENTS

TABLE OF FIGURES

Chapter One

The Need for Breast Health Information

A great deal of information is available on how to examine the breasts and look for a "lump." Women are aware of the importance of bringing a suspicious "lump" to the attention of their health care provider immediately.

Most women are informed on the unhealthy breast statistics and no doubt harbor a conscious or unconscious fear that she may enter the increasing number of those statistics.

The picture painted for women at present in order to maintain healthy breasts is to:

◆ Do monthly breast exams

◆ Stop smoking

◆ Eliminate caffeine

◆ Reduce dietary fat

◆ Wait and hope you don't develop a suspicious "lump."

You *need* to be educated about your breasts and how to keep those breasts healthy. This knowledge will assist you to take charge of your life and be responsible for your overall healthy status.

A woman's breasts are a symbol of femininity, beauty, and nurturing. As a symbol of femininity, which in turn represents the feeling or emotional part of life, the breasts are an integral part of our emotional bodies. As such, the health of the breasts is sensitive and affected by our emotions. Perhaps no single organ, with the exception of her heart, is more responsive to a woman's every thought and feeling than is the breast.

As a symbol of beauty, the breasts have uniquely represented the feminine body in all art forms. Development from childhood into womanhood is symbolized by breast development.

Perhaps we need to distinguish between "sexual" and "feminine." There is a growing trend in advertisement, entertainment, and fashion which tries to dictate a greater importance to breast size and shape. As a result, we have breast supports, almost to the extreme of a prosthesis, to make the breast visible which, at the same time, cause dangerous decreases in the circulation to and from the breasts. The use of surgery and various implants are also part of the "thing to do," all of which offer an unhealthy model for women.

Femininity is distinguished by the beauty of the woman within radiating to the woman without, through love. Femininity defined by the size of breasts is a growing, imposed trend having moral and health influences which will necessarily have to be dealt with.

The feminine Body-Temple has the ability, through nursing the newborn, to offer health protection through antibodies and nourishment for the developing infant. To have or to nurse a baby is a choice; this does not denote whether or not we are feminine.

Any threat to our unique feminine role has the potential of negatively affecting breast health. The mind/ brain does not discriminate between an imagined and a real threat, and our bodies respond to our perception of danger. Breast health appears to be an increasingly significant monitor for feminine health.

The health or wholeness of a woman is a reflection of lifestyle, our perception of reality, and our ability to joyfully fulfill our role as a woman—as we perceive it. The need now is to assume self-responsibility and take necessary actions.

Uterine cancer, once the highest cause of death due to cancer in women is, at the present time, the lowest cause of death due to cancer in women. The credit for this dramatic change goes to pap smears and early treatment.

It is my belief that a growing number of women do not want to live in subconscious fear that they may become statistics, but want to become knowledgeable, active participants in their own health. Without knowledge and alternatives, whether consciously or subconsciously, you feel there are no choices, nothing to be done that could make a difference. This belief leads to a feeling of hopelessness and a giving up of your God-given attribute of choice.

As we progress toward the 21st century, we will move from detection to prevention. Health is the natural state of your body and all body processes function in an active equilibrium, or balance, to maintain that health. Our responsibility is to become knowledgeable, active participants in a healthy lifestyle. One based on the Laws of Health which are God's Laws.

Chapter Two

The Symphony of Your Beautiful Body-Temple

I *AM" the Light that lighteth every man that cometh into the world."*

"The body is the Temple of the most high living God"

The Holy Bible

"It is highly dishonorable for a reasonable soul to live in so divinely built a mansion as the body she resides in, altogether unacquainted with the exquisite structure of it."

Robert Boyle 1627-1691

If we truly believe that the body is the Temple of God, then surely we want to know how to keep it clean, beautiful and functioning perfectly. In this book, we will not go into the concept of the "symphony" of the Body-Temple in any depth. It is important, however, to become aware that no cell, organ or system of the body operates independently of any other cell, organ or system. For this reason, breast health cannot be considered separately from the rest of the body.

A truly beautiful body, externally, is the outpicturing of the harmonious working relationship between ev-

21

ery cell, organ, and system in the body and all life. This harmony, or the collective harmonics, produces musical tones which blend together in a symphony of health. Although we cannot audibly hear this symphony, we experience its effect.

When lack of perfect functions inharmonious tones begin in one organ, let's say the colon or liver as an example, then like a squeaky violin section it affects every other organ *and* the overall symphony and health of the Body-Temple.

We can *never* have just an unhealthy breast! When signs of an unhealthy breast have been neglected until they are physically evident, many organs of the body are involved and need attention and assistance.

As we take actions to improve our breast health, we are improving our overall health. A rewarding benefit is that we are *reversing* the degenerative process beginning in the whole body. We are reversing the aging process.

Chapter Three

The Healthy Breast Versus The Congested Breast

THE HEALTHY BREAST

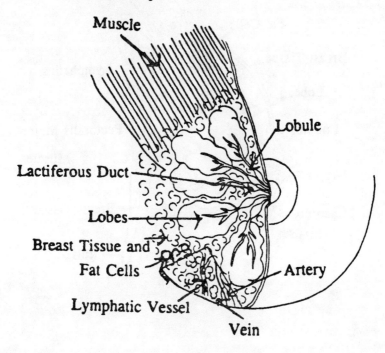

Pectoralis Major

Muscle

Lobule

Lactiferous Duct

Lobes

Breast Tissue and

Fat Cells

Artery

Lymphatic Vessel

Vein

Figure 1:   **The Healthy Breast**
           Cross-section—Front view

Important points to remember:

1.   The breast is very vascular, having an
     abundant blood and lymphatic supply.

2.   The breast has a "housecleaning system"
     called the lymphatic system.

3.   Muscles beneath the breast can affect
     breast circulation.

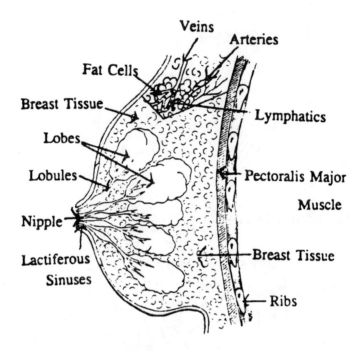

Figure 2:   **The Healthy Breast**
              Cross-section—Side view

1.   The breast tissue is divided into sections
     like spokes of a wheel or a grapefruit—
     coming off from the nipple.

2.   The breast lies against the ribs.

3.   The muscles beneath the breast are im-
     portant to breast health.

THE LYMPHATIC SYSTEM:
THE HOUSECLEANING SYSTEM
OF THE BODY

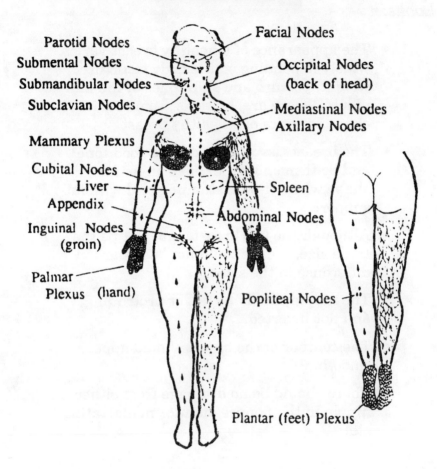

Figure 3:   Lymphatic Vessels and Lymph Nodes

Note the increased numbers of lymphatic vessels and nodes in and around the breast area as compared to the rest of the body.

HOW A HEALTHY BREAST
LOOKS AND FEELS

Looks:

♦ The appearance of a healthy breast varies
  widely depending on the body structure,
  weight, posture and skin tones of the individual. There are, however, some basic
  characteristics of a healthy breast.

♦ The breast tissue should have good tone
  and be firm enough to have an artful
  shape when viewed standing and without
  support.

♦ Although the two breasts may not be the
  same size, there should not be a marked
  difference in the size.

♦ The nipple should be flat or protruding
  and not inverted.

♦ The contour of the breast should appear
  smooth.

♦ There should be no drainage from either
  nipple in the nonpregnant or nonlactating
  state.

Feels:

Each breast should be:

♦ Soft, pliable, and with no obstructing congestion or accumulation of lymph fluid
  with debris which can be felt between

your finger and ribs as you press the breast tissue inward towards the ribs.

♦ Free of tenderness, soreness or pain in the breast tissue or in the surrounding tissue—including the region in front of or underneath the under arm (axilla).

♦ No temperature difference in any area of the breast tissue.

♦ No enlarged lymph nodes between the breasts (mediastinal nodes), underneath the collar bone (subclavicular nodes), or underneath the arms (axillary area nodes).

♦ No tenderness underneath the breasts.

♦ No lumps, no matter how small, in either breast.

THE CONGESTED BREAST

The word "congestion" is used to describe any ob-
struction in the free flow of the circulatory systems of the
breast. This includes the arterial and venous blood flow
and the lymphatic flow (the Body-Temple cleaning system).

It is called the lymph system. When it—and your
circulatory system—slows down and becomes sluggish
and congested, we could compare the results to a traffic
jam. In a congested state the cells of your breasts cannot
receive the nutrition and oxygen which should be brought
to them by healthy, free-flowing blood. Also, blood return-
ing from your breasts to your lungs and heart by the venous system is slowed down and laden with excess toxins.
The lymphatic system is overloaded and waste products
remain in those breast tissues and lymph nodes.

The following is a list which contributes to breast
congestion. Each will be discussed separately for a clearer
understanding:

- Lack of high oxygen nutritional foods.

- High protein diet.

- High fat diet.

- Unhealthy eating habits, including im-
  proper chewing of food.

- Excessive salt and sugar.

- Food combining which contributes to poor
  digestion—combining vegetables and
  fruits at the same meal.

- Habitual irregular breathing habits.

- Unhealthy brassieres.
- Backpacks which are binding and restrictive.
- Heavy purses with shoulder straps.
- Mental and emotional stress.
- Prolonged grief, not necessarily the loss of a loved one.
- Congested, poorly functioning colon.
- Irregular menstrual periods—could indicate a hormone estrogen imbalance and/or retention of toxins.
- Poor posture.
- Excessive tension in neck muscles.
- Poor self image.
- Lack of regular exercise—inactivity.
- Caffeine—including black tea and soft drinks.
- Alcohol.
- Smoking.
- High estrogen levels—from medication or foods.
- Drugs.
- Food additives which are toxic to the body.
- Fluorescent lights.

♦ High exposure to extra low frequencies (ELF)—from computers, electric blankets, TV, telephone, electric typewriters, etc.

♦ Not enough regular sunlight.

♦ Internal conflict—a conflict between what you feel is right for you (beliefs) and what you do (action).

♦ Obesity—20 percent over normal body weight.

♦ Confused, chaotic, or unorganized lifestyle.

♦ Procrastination, lack of goal setting and achievement.

♦ Lack of joy.

♦ Lack of hope.

♦ Lack of forgiveness.

♦ Lack of enough Love—of God, of ourselves—of others.

Note: The above list is not necessarily listed according to the importance of each factor.

Above all other causes, when we consciously begin to deal with forgiveness and love, then we come into a healthier state in our thoughts and feelings. We create an environment within and around ourselves that causes us to desire a healthier lifestyle, and a more loving nature. We open new doors and attract to us those persons, books, seminars, and support systems which assist us to bring about the needed changes.

Knowledge is Your Key to Good Health

HEALTHY BREASTS AND OUR BODY'S DEFENSE SYSTEM

Because of its importance to breast health, we are going to concentrate first on learning more about the lymphatic system (an important part of our defense system; study Figure 3, p. 27, again).

There appears to be very little information available concerning the relationship between healthy breasts and the lymphatic system. Knowledge of the Body-Temple and experience have demonstrated a direct connection between an efficient lymphatic system and breast health.

To understand the basics of this lymphatic system, let us be very practical and use the example of a vacuum cleaner. This vacuum cleaner is a very advanced design because it has a major responsibility to help keep the inside of our body clean. Because of this very important role, this advanced vacuum cleaner has some unique features. One of the most important features is that this system is intelligent and therefore is able to adapt to many different and changing cleaning needs. It produces its own cleaning products (antibodies, T-cells, B-cells, lymphocytes, etc.) to do specific cleaning jobs. This marvelous body cleaning system has many features which appear to be automatic, but which are in reality habitually programmed. It can also take new orders from its owner's commands by thoughts (pictures), feelings, and words (verbally spoken or silent self-talk).

This Master Vacuum Cleaner can be compared to a carpet cleaner which operates with liquid cleaning fluid. The liquid cleaning fluid in the lymphatic system is called lymph. Unlike the carpet shampoo-vacuum, our lymphatic system has many holding reservoirs called lymph nodes. These lymph nodes collect debris and toxic wastes. The intelligence in the lymphatic nodes has the ability to not only collect foreign substance and toxic wastes, but also produce a detergent effect to dissolve debris or produce special cells to engulf and digest bacteria, germs, viruses, large unused protein molecules, and other toxins which have been "vacuumed" from around the body cells.

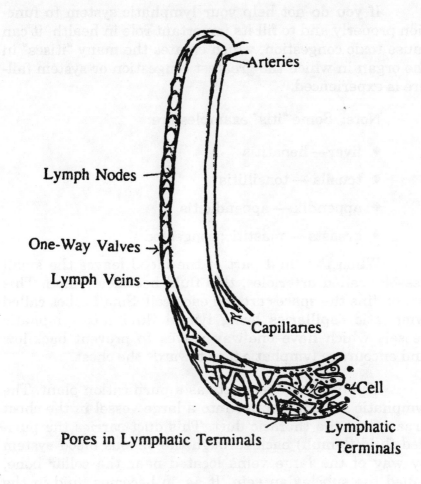

**Figure 4:   How the Lymphatic
                System Functions**

This simplified drawing represents a healthy lymphatic system. Its primary role is to keep the cell environment clean and to support cell nutrition and metabolism.

If you do not help your lymphatic system to function properly and to fill its important role in health, it can cause toxic congestion, which creates the many "itises" in the organ in which the greatest congestion or system failure is experienced.

Note: Some "itis" examples are:

◆ liver— hepatitis

◆ tonsils — tonsillitis

◆ appendix — appendicitis

◆ breasts — mastitis; congested

When the fluid part of the blood leaves the small vessels, called arterioles, this fluid becomes lymph. This lymph fills the spaces around each cell. Small tubes called lymphatic capillaries bring lymph fluid into lymphatic vessels which have one-way valves to prevent backflow and encourage lymphatic flow towards the chest.

The lymph system acts as a purification plant. The lymphatic system empties into a large vessel in the chest area called the thoracic duct. This duct carries the purified fluid (lymph) back through the venous blood system by way of the large veins located near the collar bone, called the subclavian vein. It again becomes fluid in the arterial (oxygen-carrying blood) as it leaves the left side of the heart.

LYMPHATIC SYSTEM SELF-ASSESSMENT

We are constantly monitoring our environment through our senses. Our internal environment has a feedback system from our bodies to our mind/brain and back again to provide us with information about how our body systems are functioning. Without knowledge of what this information means or how to interpret the signals, we are prone to ignore them until we are in a state of disease.

These signals, which indicate we need to be attentive and take action, are pain, soreness, heat, cold, swelling, discoloration, skin eruptions, changes in body normal functions, etc.

One method we can use to keep our systems healthy is to do a lymphatic self-assessment. Our colon, skin, kidneys, spleen, liver, lungs, and the lymphatic system have a role in helping to keep the internal systems clean. The spleen performs all the roles of the lymphatic system. Assessing the status of the lymphatic system is a good monitor for the healthy functioning of the other systems.

Refer to Figure 3, p.27, and review the lymphatic system. In our assessment we will add reflex points and areas where toxins seem likely to collect. Using the following drawing as a guide, assess the function of your lymphatic system. Remember, soreness, pain, swelling, cellulite, change in shape and/or size, etc., are all signals which need attention.

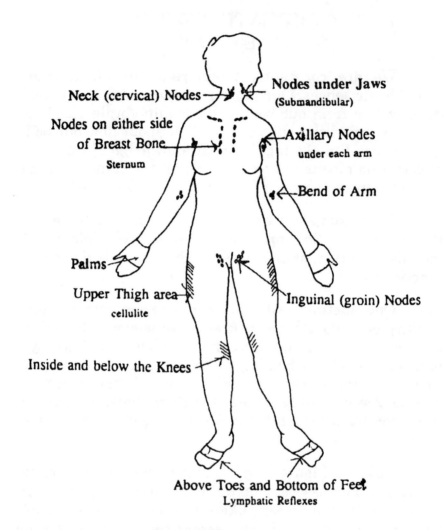

Neck (cervical) Nodes

Nodes under Jaws
(Submandibular)

Nodes on either side
of Breast Bone
Sternum

Axillary Nodes
under each arm

Bend of Arm

Palms

Upper Thigh area
cellulite

Inguinal (groin) Nodes

Inside and below the Knees

Above Toes and Bottom of Feet
Lymphatic Reflexes

Figure 5:   The Lymphatic
**   Assessment Chart**

WHY ARE WE SEEING AN INCREASE IN UNHEALTHY BREASTS?

Every decision we make concerning our lifestyle has an effect on the health of every cell in our body. The purity of the blood and its ability to carry life-giving oxygen and other necessary nutrients to the cells is affected by our lifestyle. They also affect the ability of the lymphatic system to perform its myriad housecleaning services.

The cells of your beautiful Body-Temple were so magnificently designed as to continue their specific role indefinitely—each of the cells renewing themselves at least every six months or sooner. There are, however, laws or rules which must be obeyed which allow this marvelous cell life-cycle to continue in its perfect, healthy state.

These laws or rules are found in the Ten Commandments in the Holy Bible and have been given to mankind in every major religion. Through the centuries we have never been without the availability of the knowledge of a healthy lifestyle.

Too often we have allowed ourselves to believe that we can have the freedom in life which a healthy body permits without accepting the responsibility and self-mastery required to be obedient to these simple rules which are the foundation of health.

Statistics support the fact that women are experiencing an increase in breast cancer while men are experiencing an increase in colon cancer. As individuals we each seem to have our own Achilles heel. This becomes our ability to create disease in one organ or body system which appears to manifest as a singular degenerating condition. However, as we have covered in discussing the "symphony of the Body-Temple"—no group of cells and no one organ is an island unto itself.

It would be well to review and assess the "personal check list" from the contributing factors for congested breasts.

As we will discuss in detail later, lifestyle changes should be just that—a change in the way we live. More success is experienced when we see a need to make a change, desire to make a change, and make these changes a priority for our lives.

Chapter Four

Body Organs and Systems Affecting Our Lymphatic System and Breast Health

BODY SYSTEMS AND
BREAST HEALTH

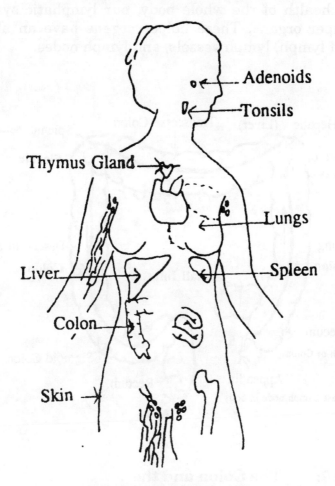

Adenoids

Tonsils

Thymus Gland

Lungs

Liver

Spleen

Colon

Skin

Figure 6: **Helper Organs to the Lymphatic System and Breast Health:**

Because our magnificent Body-Temple is wonderfully made and is a symphony of organs working together for the health of the whole body, our lymphatic system has helper organs. These helper organs have an abundance of lymph, lymph vessels, and lymph nodes.

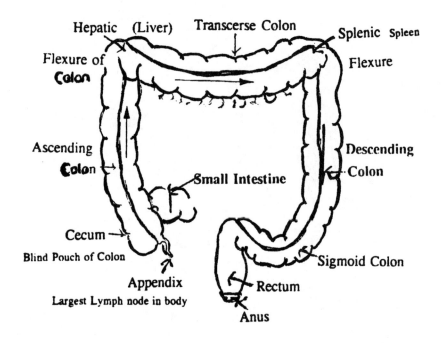

Figure 7:   The Colon and the Appendix

THE HELPER ORGANS

We will compare these helper organs to our city's water-treatment plant. If the treatment plant does not function properly or has too much waste for its ability to purify the water, the result is polluted water going out into the water distribution system. So it is with our lymphatic system. If the helper organs or "treatment plants" cannot do their job, the lymphatic system circulates toxic wastes which are dumped back into the body's circulatory system. Each helper organ which cannot rid itself of these waste products becomes a toxic waste dump and degeneration of the organ begins, which outwardly we call aging.

The Colon

Review Figure 7, p. 44 — "The Colon and the Appendix".

A good question might be, "Why would we study about the colon when our subject is breast health?"

Let us discover the relationship by looking at the colon as the drain pipe under the sink which should empty each time we put something into it. Without the role of the lymphatic system or our liquid cleansing and vacuum-cleaning system, the walls of the colon (on the inside of the sink pipe) would collect a build-up of grease, bacteria, rotting waste and would produce a foul odor resulting from the gases produced by this waste—accumulated waste.

If the colon is functioning in a healthy manner, it empties after each meal. In other words, if we eat three meals a day, we should have three colon eliminations each day. Most people believe if they have a bowel elimination every day that they are healthy. The question is, "What happened to the other two meals?" Not only do they remain in the colon; they rot, putrefy, create toxic gases and become a perfect breeding place for bacteria, viruses, atypical cells and other "small animals." This debris and toxic waste builds up on the walls of the colon and clogs up the lymphatic vacuum cleaning system for the colon. The lymph fluid becomes dirty and thick.

The accumulated debris lining the colon wall makes the colon muscles ineffective in their normal rhythmic movement intended to empty the colon's content on a regular schedule. The inside of the colon becomes a perfect setting for the creation of "sick" cells which thrive from the lack of oxygen (anaerobic) and a filthy environment.

In the colon, as well as in the small intestine, there are fingerlike projections called "villi." At the center of each villus is a lymphatic channel called a "lacteal," which is surrounded by many small blood vessels. This important role of the circulatory system to nourish and help the lymphatic system to cleanse is ineffective in a dirty, toxic colon.

Too often, instead of your colon performing its role to help cleanse your body, it becomes a toxic waste dump. The absorption of its poisonous gases and the pollution of your circulating lymphatic system affects every cell of your body—including the breasts.

The Appendix

The appendix, which was once thought to be an unimportant appendage, was often removed unnecessarily. The appendix is now known to be the largest lymph node in the body. Its location, on the "blind end" of the cecum portion of the colon is an indication of its important role to keep that portion of the colon clean. It is located at the tip of the cecum, which is the lower portion of the colon on the right side of the abdomen. An unhealthy, overworked appendix or the absence of an appendix can mean an unhealthy colon.

The Liver

As shown in Figure 5 (p.38), the liver is located on the right side of the body underneath the ribs. It is very vascular and is loaded with lymph, lymph vessels, and lymph nodes. It is the largest detoxifying organ inside the body.

The healthy liver filters and detoxifies 1,000 cc, or 1 quart, of blood every minute! After the lymph system neutralizes, dissolves, and filters the toxic waste, then the lymph is returned to the system in a state of relative purity. If the liver is congested, overworked, or not functioning properly for any reason, the blood and lymph carry "untreated and dirty" blood and lymph to other organs, such as the brain, lungs, heart, and breasts. This pollution of the blood and lymph system results in the cells of the body failing to function properly. Cell degeneration or cell aging and the production of atypical cells are given titles of diseases.

The Spleen

The spleen is the largest lymph organ in the body. It lies under the diaphragm on the upper left abdominal area (see Figure 6, p.43). One of its functions is to filter out foreign substance, as well as worn-out red blood cells, from the blood. The spleen performs all of the functions of the entire lymphatic system. It is a major defense system organ. An inefficient spleen dramatically affects our health—including breast health.

The Thymus Gland

The thymus gland is called the "master gland" of your immune system. It is located just above the heart and behind the breast bone (sternum; cf. Figure 6, p.43)

The thymus orchestrates the release of specific defense cells needed to keep us healthy and assists the lymphatic system in performing its "housecleaning" role.

The size and efficiency of the thymus gland is greatly affected by mental, emotional, and physical stress. This is why laughter has such a dramatic effect in reversing degenerative processes. A positive mental attitude, feelings of love and joy about and towards Life, have health-producing effects on the functions of the thymus gland and, therefore, on the health of the breasts.

Tonsils and Adenoids (Figure 5, p.38)

Both are lymphatic tissue and have the role of keeping the throat and nose healthy, and thus aid in preventing the spread of infection to other parts of the body.

THE COMMUNICATION SYSTEM OF THE BODY-TEMPLE

Regrettably, we know more about our washers, dryers, cars and vacuum cleaners than we do our bodies. Some of the communications by which your body tries to tell you, "something should be corrected" are:

- Loss of enthusiasm towards Life
- Tired
- Feeling "rundown"
- Sleepy during day
- Restless at night
- Lack of appetite
- Appetite cannot be satisfied
- Aches and pains
- Headaches
- Irregular menstrual periods
- Visual changes
- Skin too dry or too oily
- Hair dull, dry, or oily
- Fingernail changes—white spots, ridges, breaking or splitting easily
- Poor posture
- Constipation
- Bad breath
- Underarm odor

- ◆ Foot odor

- ◆ Less than three bowel movements a day (if eating three meals)

- ◆ Offensive urine odor

- ◆ Diminished urine output

- ◆ Enlarged lymph nodes

- ◆ Tenderness or soreness in lymph nodes

- ◆ Pain in lymph nodes

- ◆ "Heavy" breasts

- ◆ Tenderness or soreness in breasts

- ◆ "I've-never-had-large-breasts-until-I-was-forty!" syndrome (This may be partly due to obesity, but more often it is associated with very dense breast congestion.)

One or more of these messages is trying to communicate with us that we need to look for the cause and not just get rid of the effect.

Chapter Five

Assessing the Health Status Of Our Breasts

OBJECTIVES:

1. To learn more about our breasts.

2. To determine the present health status of our breasts.

3. To gather information to be used for comparison if changes occur.

IMPORTANT INFORMATION: WHAT ARE WE LOOKING FOR?

1. Normal Breasts

- ◆ Have no marked difference in size or shape

- ◆ Nipples flat or protruding

- ◆ Breast skin smooth

- ◆ Feel soft and pliable

◆ Comfortable to touch and gentle pressure

◆ No temperature differences

◆ No color differences between breasts or
  areas of a breast

2. Breasts Needing Attention

Congestion — I have defined breast congestion as a
result of the decrease or lack of normal circulation to and
from the breast tissue, any blockage in the lobes, lobules,
lactiferous sinuses or ducts, and/or any abnormal changes
in breast cell function and/or metabolism.

If you find congestion in your breast(s), the following descriptions may be helpful:

◆ Ridges — these feel like thicker tissue
  with a ridgelike surface.

◆ Cottage cheese — a softer, irregular
  lumpy area.

◆ Putty — smooth, but firmer to touch than
  the surrounding breast tissue.

◆ Pellets — tiny round formations scattered
  throughout the tissue.

◆ Balloons — tiny or small fluid-filled sacs
  or areas.

Reminder:

◆ Any "different" feeling beneath your fingers as you press towards the ribs, other

than fatty tissue held together by soft connective tissue, needs attention.

♦ Due to increased hormonal activity and increased blood circulation at the time of ovulation, menstruation, and pregnancy, some circulatory blood congestion and heaviness may be experienced. This varies from individual to individual. It is our belief that continued tenderness, soreness, or pain are signals to cleanse the breast tissue and restore normal function.

♦ A "lump" in the breast does not have to occur. Prevention is the key!

Assessment #1

Using a tape measure, measure the following areas. Date and record.

1. Measure upper arm at level of axilla (underarm).

2. Measure breasts (chest) at level of axilla (around chest).

3. Measure breast at nipple level around chest.

4. Measure just beneath breasts (exhale first).

These measurements can be done periodically as indicated.

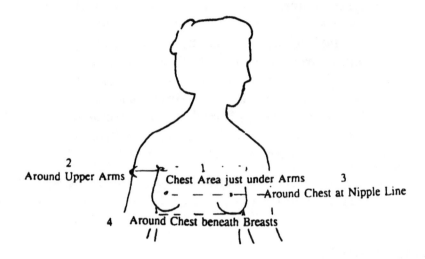

**Figure 8:   Breast Assessment and
                Arm Measurement
                Positions:**

1.   Lie on your back on a bed.

2.   Examine the left breast first.

3.   Place the left arm over your head.

4.   A pillow may be placed under your left
     shoulder to raise and flatten the breast.

5.   Lotion on the breast and examining finger
     assists in the assessment.

Assessment #2

1. Using the outer third, or pads, of your index and middle fingers, begin to assess your breast.

2. Begin at the area around the nipple and move in a circular motion, pressing inward towards the ribs.

3. Assess all the breast tissue, including about two inches beyond where you normally consider the breast tissue to end.

4. At the outer edge of the breast, near the underarm, continue to assess the tissue, including all the tissue under the arm (axilla). Congested extra breast tissue in this area, or congested lymph nodes need attention. You may shift your shoulders slightly to the right to improve your assessment.

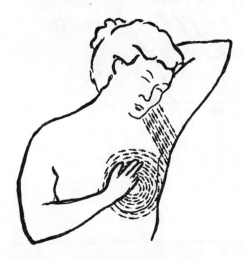

Figure 9:   Assessment #2

Assessment #3

1. Following the pattern of the lobes of the breast (refer to Figure 1, p.25), begin at the nipple area and press gently but firmly towards the outer edge of the breast and continue out for about two inches.

2. After you assess the outermost tissue area, assess inward towards the nipple.

3. Continue until all breast tissue is assessed.

Note: Refer to Figures 1 (p.25) and 2 (p.26). There are 12-15 lobes in each breast. Basically you are assessing each of these lobes.

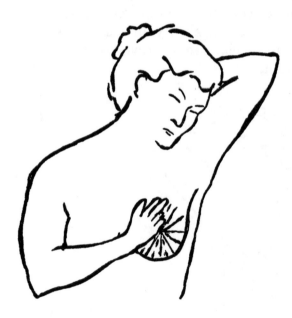

Figure 10: Assessment #3

Assessment #4

1.   Moving in a pattern perpendicular to the shoulders, begin a systematic assessment starting at the breast bone (sternum).

2.   Assess in upward lines towards the collar bone and downward towards the diaphragm.

3.   Continue to assess until all areas are covered, including two inches beyond where breast tissue is normally considered to extend.

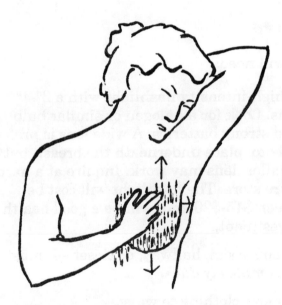

Figure 11: Assessment #4

Note: Repeat assessment on the other breast.

Assessment #5

In bathtub or shower, a wet, soapy hand and breast can be helpful in assessment.

1.   In a bathtub, sit in a semireclining position and assess as previously described.

2.   In a shower, use the hand on the same side as the breast to be examined to support the breast, if needed. If this is done, complete the assessment by raising that arm above the head and go through each assessment.

Assessment #6

You will need:

◆ A high-intensity flashlight with a 3"-4" lens. Look for a halogen or similar bulb and strong batteries. A wide lens is preferable to place underneath the breast, but a smaller lens may work. Inquire at a hardware store. The flashlight will cost between $15-$20 and will be a good health investment.

◆ A dark room, hallway, or closet—it must be *completely dark.*

1.   Remove clothing to waist.

2.   Go into dark area.

3.   Place flashlight underneath breast. Turn flashlight on and illumine breast tissue. Gently press breast down towards the

light. Move flashlight, if necessary, to illumine all areas. Healthy breasts should appear as soft pinkish tissue with no dense or dark areas—even in the larger blood vessels.

4. If the light does not illumine every area of the breast, one of several reasons should be considered.

♦ The breast is obese and too dense to illumine.

♦ The lymphatic system is clogged up.

♦ The breast circulatory system and tissue is congested.

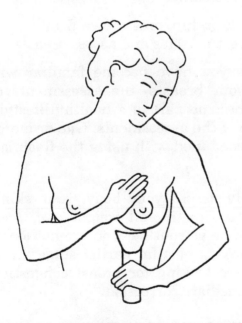

Figure 12:   Assessment #6

Assessment #7

1. Remove clothing to waist.

2. Stand before a mirror with arms at sides.

3. Assess breasts for size and shape. Note any unusual change in size or contour.

4. Look for any "dimpling" of the skin.

5. Assess nipples for inversion or drainage.

6. Pass your right hand over each breast, note any change in temperature between the two breasts.

7. Raise arms above head and repeat the above assessments.

8. Place hands on hip, press down firmly, tighten chest muscles and assess breasts.

Note: Once you have become familiar with the health status of your breasts, the assessments can be done quickly and become part of a healthy lifestyle. You can do one or more of the assessments. One or more using touch and feeling combined with using the flashlight is a good idea.

You routinely assess your body, your skin, hair, eyebrows, fingernails, teeth and weight, etc. Assessing your breasts should be as routine. You are not looking for a lump. You are looking at a far earlier stage than when lumps form. You are looking for breast congestion that needs your own immediate correction.

It can become as routine as stepping on the scales, noting a skirt is too tight, or your feet are swollen. Each is a signal to pay attention and take appropriate action.

Knowledge, prevention through awareness, and a healthy lifestyle—each defines the women of the '90's—accepting responsibility for her world.

If you disregard weight gain or a "twingy" tooth, you assume responsibility for your health status. Ignoring your breast health status is as irresponsible as ignoring these signals. I think it's rather delightful to see a clear illumination of your breasts. It's an "all clear" signal that takes about five minutes at home!

Breast Assessment Record:

A weekly or monthly breast health record may be helpful as you change to a more healthy lifestyle. After you are more knowledgeable about health and are practicing a more healthy lifestyle, a written record is not necessary.

Depending on your breast health status, breast assessment and recordings may be done on a weekly or monthly basis. Set a regular date to do these, preferably after the menstrual cycle, and mark your calendar.

An example of your record could look as follows:

Date:_____   Left Breast   Right Breast

Ridges:

Cottage Cheese:

Putty:

Pellets:

Balloons:

Notes:

Chapter Six

Restoring the Breast Section of Our Body-Temple

*I*n restoring a home, a treasured piece of furniture or a priceless piece of art, we think in terms of restoring them to their original beauty and function. How much more priceless is our Body-Temple which cannot be replaced and which was intended to be the Temple of God in which our life resides—beautiful and healthy.

As in any efficient housecleaning plan, or restoring plan, we begin by cleaning the larger areas first. We may need to scrape paint and remove wallpaper, and then end the cleaning with the smallest detail.

Likewise in each of your breasts, you first loosen up the clogging debris, then increase the ability of your natural vacuum cleaning system and finally assist your cells towards their healthy functions.

The following self-help information should be individualized to meet the needs you found in your breast and lifestyle assessment.

◆ Breast congestion does not happen overnight, and often has been accumulating for ten years or more.

67

- ◆ Your program needs to be used with wisdom, patience and persistence.

- ◆ Care of your breasts should be done with love and art—never be harsh or forceful.

- ◆ Never massage the breasts or "waltz" the lymph system to the point where you experience pain.

- ◆ Soreness and tenderness are not unusual with breast congestion, but will subside with a diligent program of helping yourself.

CLEANING THE LARGE AREAS FIRST

Colon Hygiene: (Refer again to Figure 7, p.44)

The colon has been referred to as the "drain underneath the sink." If the drain is sluggish, lined with grease and debris, and we continue to put waste in the sink, it will stop up and overflow. In beginning our larger housecleaning task, the colon needs to be cleansed by us, or by someone else who has expert knowledge of this system. You might be surprised what the following could do for your colon:

1.   An improved nutritional plan.

2.   Adequate pure water intake—a minimum of 8 glasses each day.

3.   Exercise—including abdominal exercises.

4.   Reducing stress, eliminating stressors or changing our perception of stressors.

5.   Responding to the urge to eliminate.

6.   Setting a regular time to eliminate.

7.   Becoming aware, if you do silent self-talk
     of "I'm in a hurry" or "I don't have time",
     that the body, and particularly the colon,
     believes this and responds accordingly.

8.   Forgiving yourself and others—holding on
     to negative feelings results in holding on
     to colon garbage also.

You might be amazed at the amount of garbage and
weight we can carry around in the colon.

For further information and assistance, there are
many good books on the market; or you can consult a
health professional—a health educator, a health facilita-
tor or colon hygienist.

LOOSENING UP BREAST DEBRIS

Breast Massage

Using the same position as with your assessment,
semi-lying down in the bathtub or standing in the shower;
wet the breasts and soap the hand opposite the breast you
will be examining.

◆ Begin by using the index and middle fingers to massage the nipple area in a circular motion, gently pressing inward
   towards the ribs.

◆ Continue this circular massage until you
   have covered the entire breast area, including underarm breast tissue if you

have tissue there, and have stimulated
the lymph nodes in that area.

◆ Repeat the massage several times.

◆ Now, use your whole hand to massage the
breast.

◆ Repeat on the opposite breast.

Water Breast Massage

A shower massage can be used very effectively to
stimulate the circulation of blood and lymph in the
breasts. Care should be taken to protect the nipple by covering it with your fingers. The rhythmic pulsation of the
warm water flowing through the shower massage heads
can be slowly moved in a circular motion around the
breasts, underneath the arms, and down the lymph nodes
from underneath the jaw down either side of the neck towards the large veins in the area of the collar bones.

The shower massage can also be effective in stimulating the entire lymphatic system (Refer to Figure 3,
p. 27) The shower massage should begin at the extremi-
ties—feet and hands—and move slowly towards the chest
area and the large vessels near the collar bones.

The water massage is a type of hydrocleansing. It
can not only be helpful to maintain breast health, but also
supports the flow of your lymphatic system and aids your
skin in its role of being the body's largest detoxification,
or cleansing, system.

"Waltzing" the Lymph

This technique is done to assist your lymphatic system to perform more efficiently, so it can cleanse your breast cells and help dissolve or carry away toxic substances and debris. A waltz rhythm is used because it is the natural rhythm of a healthy body. A waltz tape or record will enhance the effectiveness of this exercise.

POSITION: Same as for assessment or massage.

LEFT BREAST:

1. Using the index and middle finger of your right hand (the ring finger may also be used if more comfortable), begin to gently tap out a waltz rhythm of *hard, soft, soft* on the neck lymph nodes. (Study Figure 3, p. 27, to review the location of these lymph nodes.) It is extremely important to follow the *hard, soft, soft* rhythm, as the opposite beat, which is soft, soft, hard, will negatively affect the lymphatic flow and the health of the cells.

    Note: The *soft, soft, hard* would give the same effects as rock music, which adversely affects health—mentally, emotionally, and physically. This beat is opposite to the rhythm of the body system and creates inharmony, maladjustment of the spine and cell degeneration.

2. Continue waltzing the lymph nodes and lymph vessels downward towards the collar bone where the lymphatic system empties into the neck veins.

3. Using the same waltz rhythm, begin tapping at the inner surface of the bend in the left arm. Move upward and over to the neck vein area. Repeat on right arm.

4. Move to the underarm (axilla), giving special attention to the area of lymph nodes adjacent to the breast. Waltz the lymph nodes and vessels towards the neck veins.

5. The lymph nodes on either side of the breast bone need special attention. Using the waltzing rhythm, begin at the lower portion of the breast bone and continue upward and around the breast in a circular pattern out towards the left arm. Continue this circular lymph waltzing until you cover the nipple area.

6. Reverse this pattern, moving outward from the nipple area until you arrive at the outer edge of the breast where the lymph empties into the neck vein.

7. Repeat the same lymph waltzing on the right breast using the left fingers.

8. This lymph waltzing may be done daily.

Note: you may need to support or lift the breast up as you waltz the lymph system in order to cover all areas and stimulate drainage.

"Lymphatic Waltzing" for the General Lymphatic System

Using the same method as for waltzing the lymph vessels in the breast, take the index and middle fingers and, beginning at the feet, do a "lymphatic waltz" on the major lymph vessels as they follow the blood circulatory system. Remember, a waltz tape or record is very helpful and the symphony of the body responds to its own natural rhythm.

BRAS AND BREAST CONGESTION:

Tight, binding bras contribute to stagnation of blood circulation and lymphatic flow in the breasts and therefore affect cell health.

Bras with wire supports not only increase congestion, but act as an antenna to collect extra low electromagnetic frequencies (from T.V's., microwave ovens, telephones, electric blankets, etc.) which have an adverse effect on health.

Bras with plastic or other "boning" materials add extra pressure, decrease circulation and increase breast congestion.

Bras for Healthy Breasts Should:

1. Support the breasts without binding.

2. Be large enough to support all the breast tissue.

3.   Be constructed so that the elastic will
     easily expand and contract with breath-
     ing.

4.   The shoulder straps should be comfortable
     and not compressing. Shoulder strap
     marks should not be markedly evident
     when bra is removed.

5.   Selection of a bra is very individual and
     should be chosen to support—not bind the
     breasts. Careful attention should be given
     to not restricting the blood and lymph cir-
     culation at the outer areas near the un-
     derarms.

Note: Purses with shoulder straps should not be
heavy and carrying should be alternated between the two
shoulders.

Backpack straps can restrict circulation in the
breasts.

Baby carriers (papoose type) and some front carrying pouches can bind the breasts.

The Breath of Life:

We can survive for only a short period of time without oxygen. Oxygen is needed in the life process of every
cell of our body.

Although breathing is under the so-called automatic portion of our nervous system, it is one of the systems
with which we interfere most. To test this out, the next
time you are in heavy traffic or are listening to an un-

pleasant phone conversation, observe if you are holding your breath.

Stress is often responded to by "breath holding" and this soon results in irregular breathing patterns as a matter of habit.

What effect does this have on our health? A few of the roles which our breathing performs for us are:

1. The cerebral-spinal fluid (our nerve fluid) has no pump of its own and depends on rhythmic, balanced breathing to pump this life-giving fluid to every organ and cell of our body.

2. The breath provides oxygen which is a vital nutrient in every life-giving process of the healthy body.

3. Our breathing patterns affect cell respiration and therefore cell metabolism.

4. Our breath acts as a suction pump for the lymphatic system. Expiration creates an increased pressure which increases the vacuum cleaning effect of our lymphatic system.

Breathing Exercises:

Do these at least daily; the balanced, rhythmic pattern will soon become a habit.

Goal: To teach methods of conscious control breathing through specific exercises to restore energy balances.

Preparation:

1. Select a well-ventilated room or go outside (if air is clear).

2. During the exercises, focus your attention on "LIGHT" entering into your body as you inhale. The focus of your attention is extremely important.

3. You may sit, stand, or lie down.

Balanced Breathing:

Principle: On each inspiration, pause (hold) expiration, and pause (hold), there must be an even count. Use autogenic phrases (of even word count) on each of the four phases. An autogenic phrase is positive self-talk. It is a statement beginning with first person—present tense. Example: I am in perfect health = 6 counts.

1. Place your finger on the side of the right nostril and, as you close the right side of the nostril, breathe in air on the left side. Visualize Light coming into the body and "mentally say" an autogenic phrase of an even count (4 - 6 - 8 - 10 - 12, etc.).

2. As you continue to hold the right nostril closed, continue to visualize the Light entering the body and mentally repeat the same autogenic phrase.

3. Switch your finger to the left nostril and as you hold it closed, exhale through the right nostril.

4. Continue to visualize Light expanding throughout the body as you repeat the autogenic phrase during the "hold" phase.

5. Hold the left nostril closed as you inhale through the right nostril. Visualize the Light entering into the body as you mentally repeat the autogenic phrase.

6. Repeat as in step two.

7. Continue to repeat this balancing breathing as long as you can do it comfortably.

Remember: What your attention is on—you become.

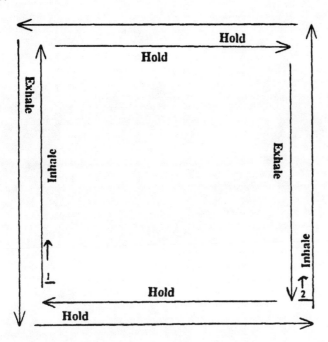

Figure 13:   Diagram of Balanced Breathing

Chapter Seven

Nutrition

*I*n school, most of us were taught about the four food groups. With closer and more informed analysis, these turn out to be representative of four major food industries.

Foods were originally categorized into three main groups, which were proteins, fats (lipids), and carbohydrates. With the growing food industries, the four categories were made and much emphasis was placed on the need for high protein intake.

More recent nutritional information has encouraged an increase in complex carbohydrates (foods containing protein, lipids, and carbohydrates) which are found in vegetables, fruits, grains, nuts and seeds and a decrease in fat and protein.

If we eat food for its nutritional value, to give us energy and provide nutrients for our body cells, it seems questionable that this can be found in dead flesh. The high intake of meat in America has been linked to the degenerative diseases. Also, meat and eggs, with their artificially added hormones, could no doubt add to a high hormonal level, causing breast changes.

A high intake of protein (more than 20%) congests the lymphatic system.

Oxygen as a life-giving nutrient has been identified by Stephen A. Levine, Ph.D., and is supported by a great deal of other research. We talk about live foods, but we are really talking about the amount of oxygen and life-giving nutrients those foods make available to your cells. The amount of oxygen or life-energy in a food provides the spark of life necessary for converting the potential energy in the food into useable chemical energy. Living complex carbohydrates are high oxygen nutrient foods for you and your breasts. The riper the food is when it is harvested, the fresher we can obtain it and the better we can preserve its life-energy, the more "nutrition" we obtain from food.

The efficiency of our defense system depends on having adequate amounts of oxygen available to the cells. Yeast infections, cancer cells, viruses and bacteria develop, grow, and multiply in an anaerobic (oxygen-deprived) environment.

Caffeine drinks, coffee, black teas, meats—especially red and pork—white sugar and fats create an acid condition in the cells. Oxygen is used to help neutralize the acid and is therefore not available for normal cell metabolism and health. Dense food and those high in fats—i.e., steaks and other meats, cheese, potato chips, ice cream, etc.—require extra oxygen and this results in less oxygen being available for the cells.

A diet high in fats means you are probably consuming large quantities of fat-soluble toxins found in food—pesticides, herbicides, etc. Like diets high in protein, diets high in fat have been associated with degenerative diseases. Oxygen is again required to metabolize

food—pesticides, herbicides, etc. Like diets high in protein, diets high in fat have been associated with degenerative diseases. Oxygen is again required to metabolize these, and a healthy lymphatic system is needed to remove these from the body.

The average American eats 120 grams of protein daily. This is 100 grams in excess of what the body needs for healthy tissue. This excess protein overtaxes the kidneys, increases blood acidity, and acts as a toxin in the body cells. A nutritional lifestyle change would call for a planned reduction of protein to 20% of our daily food intake.

A health-producing nutritional program would consist of:

- ◆ Complex carbohydrates   60%
- ◆ Protein   20%
- ◆ Fat (Lipids-Oils)   20%

(Most of this can be gotten in the complex carbohydrates.)

Note: Complex carbohydrates are found in vegetables, fruits, grains, seeds (sprouted), nuts (sprouted).

Basic guidelines for improving nutrition have to do with each link in the chain, from growing the food until it is eaten.

- ◆ *Growing of food* is beyond the control of
  most of us; however, it will be an informed
  public who will eventually demand
  changes in the way food is grown and in
  the pesticides and chemicals used which
  eventually end up in our bodies.

and grains will improve nutrition. Fresh
foods are generally our best choice, except
when processes such as waxing, gassing,
etc. are used to keep them in their "fresh"
state. In some instances, frozen vegetables
may be our better choice if the food lends
itself to freezing. Frozen vegetables have
usually been picked ripe (where more nutrients have been produced) and frozen
quickly.

As a general guideline, the order of
selection of foods for their nutritional value would be: fresh, frozen, dried, and
canned. Grains which have not been denatured or separated from the whole grain
are your best choice. Examples of denatured grains are polished white rice, white
flour (which has had the bran and nutrients removed, has been bleached and has
had only some of the vitamins and minerals replaced). Pasteurized and homoge-
nized dairy products are another example
of denatured food. It is the belief of a number of health educators that milk should
not be a part of the diet after the baby's
first teeth are through.

Decaffinated coffee, tea, and soft drinks
may be more harmful than the "real"
thing. Sugar substitutes may be more
harmful than sugar and natural drink
sweeteners.

◆ Food preservatives, dyes, additives, and
processing should all be considered in the
selection of the best food available. Disre-

garding the quality of the food we select or becoming a food fanatic both seem to be out of balance.

◆ *Storing foods* should be given careful consideration, to preserve their nutritional value. Since "freshness" or retention of nutrients, including oxygen, color and texture, is very important, fresh fruits and vegetables should be purchased in amounts in which they can be eaten in three days. Each food should be stored to preserve the fresh state as much as possible. Whether the food requires a dark, dry, airtight, cold or moist environment—each food should be stored properly.

◆ *Preparing foods* in a manner to preserve as much nutritional value as possible is important. If we like the taste of a food that is overcooked, then we should consider it to have very little nutritional value left for our cells. A guideline for preserving nutrients in preparation is:

Fresh and raw (this does not mean we should eat all raw food)

Steamed

Sauteed (lightly stir fry)

Baked—broiled

Boiled (saving liquid for soups or sauces if not served with or in the food)

Fried. (Avoid as much as possible.)

◆ *Cooking utensils* are important because
they can become part of what we eat. The
following list is a guide for utensil selection:

Stainless steel (heavy)

Pyrex

Iron

Enamel (no chips or cracks)

Aluminum cookware is hazardous to health!
Small amounts of aluminum are leached out during the
cooking process. This amount of aluminum, added to the
amounts we get in foil-wrapped food, aluminum canned
drinks, etc., adds up to toxicity which speeds up cell aging
and degenerative diseases.

◆ *Food combinations* are important in meal
planning. If you are unfamiliar with proper food combining, get a food combining
chart or card. Basically, one of the most
frequent problems in food combining is
the serving of fruits and vegetables at the
same meal. These foods require different
digestive juices and one or both are not going to be properly digested. This not only
affects our digestive system, but deprives
our bodies of needed nutrients.

◆ *Color combinations* are extremely important in planning meals. Each food color
represents the nutrients available in the
food. The colors of food combinations make
the meal appetizing and eye-appealing,
and gives a balance to the nutrients in the

different foods. An example of a highly
nutritional salad is to put as many different colored vegetables in a salad as possible—make a rainbow salad!

◆ *Preparing the eating environment* in order
that the meal will be in a pleasant atmo-
sphere, quiet talk (no problems discussed),
non-hurried and without interruptions (no
phone answering) is important to a
healthy lifestyle.

◆ *Serving the food* as attractively as possible
is important to appetite and preparation
for digestion.

◆ *Final food preparation* is asking the food
to be Blessed when we have done all the
above to the best of our ability, even if
canned food was the best we could provide. It is my belief that, when the food is
Blessed with an understanding of the true
purpose of Blessing the food, that the food
is changed nutritionally and gives us the
nutrients we need.

What We Eat: What's Eating Us

The truly nutritional value of our food, how we select it, store it, prepare it and serve it is extremely important. *The person who is eating the food is equally
important!*

The most nutritional food eaten by someone who is
emotionally upset or under excess stress cannot be properly digested. Undigested food acts as a toxin. Most of us
have had the experience of being ready to eat a meal and

then had a stressful conversation or phone call and immediately lost our appetite. This, in reality, is a protective mechanism and a signal that it is not a good time to ignore the signal and eat the meal.

The person who is habitually "upset," stressed, or negative in her feelings no longer receives the protective signal and food is put into a digestive system which is not prepared to receive it. The results are indigestion and decreased colon activity, resulting in constipation. The opposite can occur—that of irritable colon, which can result in diarrhea. In any case, the food has had to be handled by digestive fluids which have been chemically changed and/or decreased. Digestive enzymes are not produced in sufficient amounts to effectively assist in the normal digestive process.

Our personal preparation prior to eating a meal is as important as the food we eat. Meals are the time we physically nourish our bodies. Along with the very best food possible, we have further responsibility for our nutrition, and that is our own preparation to receive the food. An uncluttered mind and a peaceful emotional body are extremely important prerequisites for digesting and absorbing nutrients from food.

Chapter Eight

The Importance of Water

*E*ighty percent of our bodies should be composed of fluid, of which the basic component is water. With the pace of today's schedules, most of us do not habitually drink enough water to provide this necessary fluid for healthy body processes.

Lack of enough water taken into our bodies at regular intervals and on a daily basis affects every cell and all body systems. Studies have shown the negative effects of low water intake on our ability to learn and it has been identified as a factor in premature labor. The more subtle effects of low water intake take place on the cellular level and adversely affect normal cell metabolism. Many agree that fluids should not be taken along with a meal because they dilute the digestive fluids; however, water taken thirty minutes before or after a meal is essential. If your water intake is low, your body, in its effort to obtain more fluid, will absorb water from your colon and this contributes to constipation.

One function of the liver is to filter our blood; in fact, it should filter about a quart of blood every minute. An adequate amount of water intake assists in cleansing your blood. Your liver is also responsible for fat metabolism. Without enough water intake your liver is busy filtering waste that should be filtered by your kidneys, and thus your liver won't burn fat as is should.

The main water filtering plant of the body is the kidney. Not drinking enough water or taking medications to forcibly rid the body of retained fluids are both confusing to the body cell intelligence. The cells will interpret a decrease in water as a threat of dehydration and will begin to retain fluid in the spaces around the cells. If we have an excess salt intake, even more fluid is retained. Using a medication—a diuretic to force the cells to release fluid—also robs the body of necessary minerals that are needed for proper cell functioning and health.

If you are retaining fluid, and you increase your fluid intake as I show you, the result is the loss of excess body fluid and an improvement of cell metabolism. The drinking of at least eight glasses of pure water on a daily basis affects every system of our bodies, including the very important lymphatic system, the kidneys, liver, and the health of our skin. Drinking adequate amounts of water on a regular basis is important to the health of every cell of our bodies.

In breast congestion or weight gain, most women would benefit from at least two quarts of pure water a day. At first you may feel you are drinking too much water, and you really don't desire the additional water. One reason for this is that the center in the brain responsible for thirst is easily and quickly satisfied. Many people have habitually been neglectful about drinking an adequate water intake. In this instance, the brain does not continue to give a signal of thirst except when we are actually dehydrated. To change this habit of drinking too little water, the following ideas may work well for you.

◆ Obtain a gallon of pure water; if at home, put it on the kitchen cabinet—if at work, put it under your desk or in a convenient place where you can see it and it will be easily accessible.

◆ Use a quart container with a straw and refill it with water each time you drink a quart. You may find you will drink more water when using a straw.

◆ Set a goal to drink at least two quarts a day.

Your body cells will love the internal bath; your organs will enjoy the needed fluid, your muscles will begin to tone, your skin will take on a new glow. A further advantage is that your weight will be reduced, your circulatory and excretory systems will function more effectively and your lymphatic system will do a good housecleaning job. Your general health as well as your breast health will improve with this increased amount of water intake.

Chapter Nine

Exercise and Breast Health

*M*ovement and activity are necessary for life and health. A regular exercise program should be as important in our lifestyle as eating, for both are important in maintaining health.

Congested breasts are a sign of a sedentary lifestyle. This does not mean a woman is not busy; it does mean that we can be very busy and still not exercise our body.

Some of the signs of lack of exercise are: overweight, cellulite (we notice this even on teenagers and young women—appearing as cottage cheese effect under the skin, particularly at the thighs), lack of skin tone, flabby arms and legs, enlarged knee areas, etc.

A comment we often hear is, "I never had large breasts until I was 35 or 40, and now I wear a size (or two) larger bra." Some of this may be due to increase in fatty tissue because of weight gain—and this is not healthy. Along with increased fatty tissue comes breast congestion. This results in a growing amount of toxicity in the blood, slowing down of blood and lymph fluid circulation. The breasts may even become so heavy they affect posture and the underneath breast tissue becomes even more congested.

At rest, the lymph fluid moves through its vessels at a rate of 1/16 an ounce or less each minute. During mild activity the rate increases to 3/4 ounce or more per minute. There is three times more lymph fluid in the body than blood. Vigorous exercise can increase the lymph fluid circulation to ten times that of its circulation at rest.

Let's learn about some ways to keep this fluid moving and thus increase the efficiency of our defense system—our housecleaning system—and therefore improve our health.

Walking

Walking in fresh air is the most effective overall exercise. The speed of your walking should be individualized and the length of distance or time gradually increased to your endurance. A regular walk of at least three times a week is effective and can become a part of a healthy lifestyle. Lifestyle is the key!—not just an exercise program to go on until breast congestion is no longer apparent.

Callanetics

Callanetics is a series of muscle lengthening or re-lengthening (stretching) and toning of muscles. These exercises are taught by Callan Pinckney. Callan has taught these exercises to thousands of people over the last 20 years with almost unbelievable results. She has written several books and has three video tapes to teach the beginner, intermediate and advanced student.

Without the lengthening (stretching) of muscles and the realignment of our frame (our skeleton-bones) we cannot have a beautiful Body-Temple.

Jogging

Jogging, although still popular, has many adverse effects on health. Even with the best shoes, the trauma of jogging damages the ankles, knees, kidneys (they have inadequate support for such harsh treatment) and breasts. Although there are athletic bras—these still do not protect this delicate tissue from the trauma of jogging.

Running

Running is less damaging than jogging, but, for the general population of women, is not safe for the breasts and is not an exercise most women should do regularly.

Swimming

Swimming is a very good exercise and, if it is possible for you to swim regularly, it may be your exercise of choice.

Mini-trampoline

What kind of an exercise can a woman do to help restore the Body-Temple? How can we most effectively exercise to help the most, in the least amount of time from the daily schedule, and have the greatest result for the lymphatic system?

The mini-trampoline, this seemingly simple device, is the most effective means of stimulating the general lymphatic circulation. Doing the "lymphatic exercise" on the mini-trampoline, or rebounder, creates the greatest assistance to your lymphatic vacuum cleaning system with the least amount of effort. The lymphatic vessels, or hose, have one-way valves which assist in moving toxins, excess protein, and other debris from around the cells towards their final emptying into the neck veins. The effect of overcoming gravity when your feet leave the trampoline, as you jump up for only six inches and breathe in, is to open up the lymphatic valves. Every lymphatic valve opens and encourages the upward flow of lymph fluid carrying out its housecleaning task. As your feet come in contact with the mini-trampoline pad and you exhale, the lymphatic valves close and the cells squeeze together. Toxins, excess protein and debris are squeezed out and preparation has been made for the next upward jump with the suctioning, cleaning effect of this lymphatic vacuum.

The inhaling of your breath as your feet leave the mini-trampoline pad and the exhaling of your breath as your feet touch the pad are very important, and make the exercise more effective in stimulating the lymph fluid flow. Be careful not to hyperventilate!

Lymphatic Pump Exercise

This mini-trampoline exercise is done without letting your feet leave the trampoline pad. It also incorporates inhaling as you pump—4 to 6 times, depending on your lung capacity—and then exhaling for the next 4 to 6 pumps. Keep your attention focused on LIGHT.

Note: Any good exercise program which exercises all of the body includes exercises in which toxins and debris are squeezed out, circulation in the breasts is stimulated, excess weight is reduced and your tissues are toned. Exercises in which neck, shoulder, and upper back tension is drained out are extremely important to breast health. Breast health is a result of a healthy lifestyle, which includes a regular exercise program that is effective for all body systems.

REFLEXING THE LYMPHATICS: A PASSIVE EXERCISE

It has long been known that the feet have reflex points on them which relate to each body organ and system. The charts opposite outline these points and emphasize the lymphatic stimulation areas. In massaging these areas, remember to be gentle and consistent. During or after a bath or shower is a good time to incorporate this health care stimulation into your new lifestyle.

It's a good idea to drink a glass of pure water after any exercise or reflexing. The water assists in carrying off the debris.

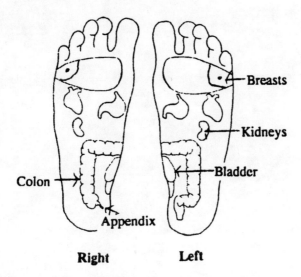

Right   Left

**Figure 14A: Reflex and Lymphatic
              Stimulation Points on the
              Feet**

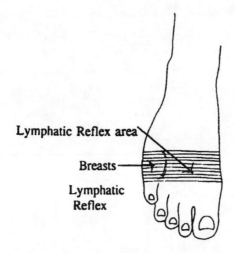

**Figure 14B: Reflex and Lymphatic
              Stimulation Points on the
              Feet**

Chapter Ten

Obesity

*O*besity and health are not synonymous! Obesity and congestion in the circulation of the breasts are synonymous! Obesity is defined as weighing 20% over normal body weight. This does not mean that women with average or below average weight do not develop poor breast health; it does mean that obesity is not healthy.

Obesity is a symptom, an effect, and is due to a variety of mental, emotional, and physical causes.

The basic steps in weight control are:

1. Desiring to lose excess weight.

2. Determining that we are overweight—not that our clothes are shrinking or that we are retaining a lot more water than usual! We must be honest with ourselves—this is a giant step!

3. Deciding we really want to "release" the extra weight we are holding onto.

4. Developing a plan to control weight which is a lifestyle change. There are self-help

107

programs as well as commercial programs
with group and/or individual support systems available. Investigate several programs and choose the one best suited to
your needs.

5. Rewards—from the beginning of your
    weight control program, decide on periodic
    rewards as you achieve your goals and *re-
    ward yourself.* Posture and self image will
    improve as you begin to feel good about
    yourself, so *plan* to reward your successes.

Note: Much has been said and written on obesity.
A plan of action and a change in the lifestyle is what is
needed.

Chapter Eleven

Posture and
Breast Health

*T*he chest, and therefore the breasts, should be the most forward portion of the body.

When thoughts get more and more negative and become energized by strong negative emotions, our bodies begin to respond. Indeed, our bodies are like computer printout sheets—they create pictures of what we think (pictures in our minds), feel, and talk about.

Every atom, cell, organ and system responds to these mind/brain master computer commands. Our attitude is reflected in our posture. The outward evidence of what goes on inside is reflected in our frame—the muscles and bones which respond in a puppetlike fashion to the quality of messages being sent to them by the nervous system. Our bodies respond by taking on an unbalanced attitude or posture. Typical responses are that the head and neck assume a forward thrust which gives the appearance that we're fighting the whole world. Another is that the head and neck are in a "laid back" position, giving the attitude that we don't care.

In breast congestion we usually see the head and neck forward and, as the attitude and posture become

111

more stressed, worried, and negative, the large muscles (pectoralis major) begin to shorten and contract. The contraction of this large muscle which lies just beneath the breasts also affects the circulation of the breasts and, in particular, the lymphatic circulation. Posture is not only an important indicator of how we see and feel about ourselves, but also of how a less than erect posture affects breast health. This is probably a good time to put your book down and carefully analyze your posture.

Stand in front of a full-length mirror. Look at yourself in front and both side views. Take both hands and push the abdomen inward—notice what happens to the breasts. Lift your head and neck in an upward, balanced, erect position with the chest slightly forward. Level the shoulders, tighten your buttocks, tilt your pelvis slightly forward and tighten the abdominal muscles. Bring both arms in a wide circle, beginning in front of your body, over the head, as far back as possible, and then let your arms hang loose at your sides. Viewing the body from the side, one should be able to draw a straight line down the side of the head, down through the earlobe, through the center of the upper arm and on downward through the center of the ankle and to the floor. This posture allows the internal organs to begin to function in their normal positions, allows you to breathe more deeply and places the body in its normal attitude or posture.

Our conscious awareness of the need to improve our posture and make the effort to be aware of how we are standing, sitting, and sleeping is an important step in improving our attitudes and self-image. Sitting and sleeping positions or postures are equally as important as standing ones. Each are indicators of how we think and feel, as well as what we talk about and the resulting actions we take.

To improve your sitting posture, select a comfortable chair that has a firm but comfortable seat cushion, supports the back so it can be slightly forward, with your feet comfortably resting on the floor. When sitting for periods of time at a desk, select a chair which can be adjusted to your individual needs.

Sleeping posture should be on the back or on either side, with the knees slightly bent in either position. Lying on the back can be made more comfortable by placing a small soft pillow under the knees. Posture is a matter of our body position or attitude 24 hours a day!

Chapter Twelve

Music and Breast Health

E *arlier* we talked about the healthy body as a symphony; each organ producing its own keynote or chord, blending with and affecting harmonics of the body systems into a beautiful symphony.

"Harmony" is a key word. Health or harmony is affected by one organ or system which is not functioning in health, or is inharmonious, the way an organ produces an inharmonious tone which in turn affects all other systems. Indeed, we never have just one organ or system out of health or harmony.

Inharmonious, discordant tones do not begin with, or in, a body organ. These negative tones are carried to the organ through the liquid in our bodies, collectively known as our emotional body. The vibrational frequencies produced by our feelings determine whether there is harmony or discord in the organs. It's easy to see that how we think and feel affects the harmony of our Body-Temple.

Sounds outside of and surrounding our bodies are of two main types—musical tones or noise; both affect our health.

Noise is discordant sound. Noise, under the guise of music, can be as addictive as drugs and just as destructive to our bodies. The destructive so-called music is rock music, in all its debilitating forms, blues and jazz. Rock music has a beat of soft, soft, hard, while music in harmony with our bodies has just the opposite rhythm of hard, soft, soft. The beat, or reversed rhythm, of rock music literally shatters the harmonies of the cells and greatly contributes to the degeneration of cells, or cell aging. Jazz so-called music has no rhythm or no definite beat and creates confusion in the cell harmonies. Blues are depressing and lower cell activity.

Our Body-Temple health is dynamically, but subversively and subtly, affected by the music we listen to by choice or which surrounds us in our various environments. Most people are aware of the high noise levels of rock so-called music and its effect on hearing. A growing number of people, taking responsibility for their health status, are becoming informed about the difference between music and noise and the effect each has on health. If you are experiencing breast congestion, music and noise are two environmental factors you should assess.

On a positive note—include singing a happy song in your new lifestyle. A happy song and stress or depression cannot occupy the same Body-Temple.

Chapter Thirteen

Unorganized Lifestyle

A *chaotic*, unorganized lifestyle is usually supported by lack of goal setting and procrastination. These habits of lifestyle are often reflected in internal confusion and the resulting negative effects on our health.

Recall how you feel in a traffic jam, as opposed to how you feel when traffic is moving freely. In the same way, mental and emotional conflicts, lack of organization and planning in our lives leads to changes in body chemistry, poor digestion, and stress which produces congestion in all body systems.

Assess how you feel when you walk into a cluttered room, sit down at a cluttered desk, or look into a disorganized closet. Does it affect how you feel, what you are able to accomplish, and the way you perceive your goals?

How do you feel mentally and emotionally when your environment is in order—is organized? Order is a law of the Universe; order in our lives internally and externally is basic to health.

As we begin to consciously access our lifestyles—develop goals, make constructive changes and put these into action—our bodies respond in a positive way. They begin to operate in harmony with our healthy life-style.

Chapter Fourteen

Emotions and Breast Health

*A*S A WOMAN THINKETH (AND FEELETH) SO SHE IS!

As creative beings of choice, we are unique in that we can think, feel and talk (either silently or in outer verbal speech) in any manner we choose. These are very powerful creative powers and, although we do choose how we use them, often our choices have become habits which seem to be automatic responses.

Our bodies do not run on automatic even though we may have been taught that they do. We may believe that we really have no responsibility for the conditions we find ourselves in nor the status of our health. It's rather a rude awakening to discover that we are responsible for running our own worlds! This leaves very little time, if any, to run anyone else! The truth is, if we spend time trying to manage, or run, someone else's world, then our attention is not on our world and things may get out of order, clog up, and begin to degenerate!

Experience with women and breast health has lead me to believe that the condition of breast congestion has to do a lot with the way you think, feel (your emotions) and how you talk to yourself and others.

125

Let's look at some powerful energies which begin to deteriorate our cells (aging), clog up our systems and, in general, change a beautiful body symphony into a screeching, noisy, clogged up, falling apart system. We will only list these and encourage you to reflect on them as you contemplate some positive lifestyle changes. We encourage you to list some feelings you may have and would like to change. Some feelings to consider are:

- fear
- doubt
- resentment
- hate
- dislike
- anger
- blaming of others
- jealousy
- limitation
- hopelessness
- guilt
- unworthness

What you think about most, what you believe is true and how you talk—all determine what is in your world and your health.

- You can choose to think positive, health-producing thoughts.

- We can choose to replace negative feelings with Love. "Love our so-called en-

emy," "Love our neighbor as ourselves."
One of the needs may be to love all Good,
the God within, above us, and around us
and in Life.

♦ We can consciously love God, with all our
   hearts.

♦ We can count to ten before negative words
  attempt to leave our mouth.

♦ Consciously talk positively—plan it and
  do it!

♦ Be grateful for life and for the privilege of
  being responsible for it.

♦ Love your Body-Temple.

STRESS, CONFLICT . . .
AND BREAST CONGESTION

Although no major negative health status occurs
overnight, we have set the stage or prepared for it over a
period of time. We have observed that the congestion in
the breasts which gets our attention is often associated
with a stressful emotional situation.

A stressful emotional crisis for many women is focused in the breasts. This could be because of the relationship of emotions to the breasts. In assisting women,
we have found that a personal emotional crisis arising out
of a conflict between what they are doing in their lives
and that conflicting with their belief system can create
breast congestion. Marital or family emotional crisis is a
stress of enough magnitude to begin to destroy the Body-
Temple, and often expresses in increased breast conges-

tion. A feeling or belief that she is no longer needed, attractive or loved can also express in noticeable breast congestion.

LOVE, JOY, HOPE, AND GRATEFULNESS

All of these are the basis for our health. I have found that the lack of these positive feelings about and towards life are often associated with the status of breast health.

Do I really Love?

Do I easily express Love?

Do others Love me?

All energy travels in a circle. If we are not loved as we would like to be—perhaps we have not loved enough.

Do I feel a joy about life; in my associations; in my work?

If this is a feeling I haven't learned or used in a while, perhaps I need to find something I can really feel joyful about.

"See" clearly the picture of whatever is a joy for you.

Feel the joy!

Note: At first it may seem unusual or awkward—something like walking on a leg that's been in a cast a long time. With practice we can become a more joyful person.

Joy turns on the energy of Life.

Joy energizes the thymus gland—which in turn operates a healthier immune system. Together these help keep our breasts healthy.

Hope means we can see and plan beyond today.

Gratefulness — practice being grateful for life, grateful for the day and grateful for all "opportunities."

Love of life, Love of the God within, above and all around us, and the Love of and to others is the *great healer emotion*! Along with the goal to change an unhealthy lifestyle to a health-sustaining one, begins the road to a feeling of self-control, being in charge of our lives, and the goal of true happiness that life was meant to be.

Chapter Fifteen

Fear and Breast Congestion

*F*ears are "tied up" in a variety of packages, some we are consciously aware of, some hidden in long-term memory, and many held in the subconscious just waiting for an opportunity to rise up to conscious awareness.

To say that we do not harbor some degree of fear concerning the health of our breasts would be denying the frequent reminders facing us in our society. Statistics of women who do not have healthy breasts, our likelihood of becoming another statistic, or a celebrity who has all of a sudden "discovered" that her breast health was in jeopardy, create conscious or subconscious fears.

The emotion of fear contracts muscles and congests the normal flow of nerve, blood, digestive and lymphatic fluids. Our bodies respond in the above reaction whether the fear is from a real or imagined threat.

Some fears which adversely affect our immune system and our health are:

- Fear of cancer of the breast
- Fear of loss of breast

- ◆ Fear of aging

- ◆ Fear of not being accepted

- ◆ Fear of not being needed—children leaving home

- ◆ Fear of loss of marriage—another woman

- ◆ Fear of no longer being attractive

- ◆ Fear of uncertainty in being fulfilled or attaining goals

- ◆ Fear of unknown—future

- ◆ Fear of death

FEAR AND LOVE CANNOT COEXIST

You can choose the emotion you want to rule your life. Here's how: make a list of the fears you are experiencing—real or imagined. Each are equally destructive. Beside each fear write down what action you are going to take to eliminate the fear. The fact that you have written each fear down has some effect on neutralizing the fear. It has brought it up to conscious awareness and it's like bringing them out of the dark and shining a light on them. This way they don't seem as fearful. And now that you are going to do something about them, they begin to become powerless. You've taken another step towards self-control, responsibility, and health!

As we enter into a period of self-responsibility through knowledge and action, we have an exciting opportunity to take control of our lives and develop a lifestyle which supports our natural state of health.

Chapter Sixteen

Forgiveness: A Basic Ingredient For Health

*T*o truly forgive ourselves and others means to replace the feeling which caused us to need to forgive with Love. When we have truly forgiven, we no longer think, feel, or talk about these negative beliefs or situations which have caused us so much stress.

Once we have brought the need to forgive up to conscious awareness, we have taken a major step. Becoming aware is important, but then we must take action. Beginning with ourselves is a good place to start. If we cannot forgive ourselves—how can we forgive others?

It's interesting that God forgives the instant we ask! Who are we not to accept that we are forgiven or that we can forgive ourselves. I have found that the lack of these two—accepting forgiveness and forgiving ourselves—are basic to weight control, overall health, and breast health.

Forgiving others takes just as much determination and practice. A subtle form of needing to forgive others comes in the form of feeling "hurt"—another word for "anger." We can only change ourselves! It's very interesting, however, that as we change ourselves—just magically others seem to change! Old "hurts" poison our bodies by

changing body chemistry. They change or slow down normal body processes. Old "hurts" congest circulation, cause
changes in cell metabolism and speed up the aging process. In other words, they begin to destroy—degenerate
the Body-Temple.

SOME IDEAS FOR FORGIVING OURSELVES AND OTHERS ARE:

Forgiving Ourselves:

Take time to make a list of any negative thoughts
and feelings you have about yourself or any negative self-
talk. Also consider the way you talk about yourself to others. Examples might be: "I always forget to do that!" "I'm
so clumsy!" "Every time I eat a piece of pie I gain five
pounds!" (A verbal command to which our body metabolism must respond!) "I can never lose weight!" "I can
never forgive myself for doing that!"

Beside each of these, write, "I forgive myself!"
Then write a positive statement to replace the old habit.
As you practice forgiving yourself and practice the new
statements, your body and world will begin almost magically to change.

Practice—Practice—Practice

Forgiving Others:

Of course we have to *want* to! The human side of us might want to hold on for dear life to old grudges, hurts, resentments, anger, dislikes, hate, blame, criticism, jealousy and all the other garbage. Never does the real Self—the God within us—want to harbor these feelings. These feelings are harming our bodies much more than they are harming anyone else! If we really want to clean house, the following ideas may be helpful:

- ◆ Make a list of people you want to forgive. Beside each name, write a feeling which you have towards them that you desire to correct. Then write down, "I forgive you and send you my Love!"

- ◆ Make another list of the same names. This time write beside each name, "I forgive you and send you my Love!"

- ◆ Burn the first list!

- ◆ At night before you go to sleep, call each name and tell them, "I forgive you and send you my Love!"

Forgiveness Is an Important Part of a
Healthy Lifestyle

Chapter Seventeen

Spiritual
Health

*T*he crises we create in our lives can be changed into *opportunities* if we choose. Often these "opportunities" offer us a chance to look, not only at making needed changes in our lifestyle, but also inside ourselves to re-evaluate our values and beliefs.

A major stressor is any difference between what we believe to be true in our hearts, what we think intellectually and how we live our lives. Often we respond to the many seeming demands of life and neglect taking the time for ourselves, to reflect, contemplate, and become consciously aware of the source of our Life. We need to become aware of our responsibility to that God-Life within us.

Taking the opportunity to assess our spiritual beliefs and determine if we are living those beliefs is the first step towards spiritual health, and ultimately our mental, emotional, and physical health.

Contemplate your answers to the following questions:

1. How do I see God?

2. How do I experience God?

143

3. What example(s) do I have for daily liv-
    ing?

4. Are there really Laws of Life to live by?

5. Does the lifestyle I live, how I take care of
    myself, and relate to others and the world
    really matter?

6. Is there Life after so-called death?

Chapter Eighteen

Taking Charge

G OAL SETTING:

Lifestyle changes require that we set goals. To set a goal we must first determine what needs to be changed.

Make a list of changes you feel you need to and desire to change.

Write a goal down in the first person, present tense, as if it is already accomplished.

The order-taker part of the brain does not know the difference between imagination and reality, it just takes orders. These orders or goals must be as clearly stated as a computer program. You must be able to see and feel yourself in the picture of the accomplished goal and be able to draw it.

Example: I weigh 130 pounds.

♦ Beneath the goal, write down specific action steps you need to take to accomplish your goal.

Examples: I exercise for 30 minutes by walking on Monday, Wednesday, and Friday at 5:30 p.m.

> I exercise on my mini-trampoline for
> five minutes every morning at 6:00 a.m.

◆ Read your goals every night before retir-
ing. You are the conductor of your body-
symphony and the master of your world.
Our body and our world respond to our
conscious or habitual orders through what
we think, feel, and silently or verbally talk
about.

◆ *Desire*—just *love* to accomplish your goal.

◆ *Determination* and persistence, in spite of
all appearances, will pay off with success.

◆ *Destination,* or goal achievement, will be
the result.

Let's review the 4-D formula for Goal Achievement:

◆ *Desire* the accomplished goal—Love it.

◆ *Decide* on what you want. Think about it,
visualize it.

◆ *Determination*—Stick with the goal and
the action items until you succeed—Ex-
pect to succeed.

◆ *Destination*—Goal accomplished! Reward
yourself! Don't depend on others for your
rewards. Decide on a reward before you
begin your goal program. When you accomplish your goal—reward yourself.

You are worth it!

DEVELOP MORE GOALS!

Developing a Healthy Lifestyle

This is not a program; it is a *process*.

It is not a one-time thing you do; it is a continual process of self-evaluation, planning, doing, achieving, and doing it all over again.

Is it worth it? Only you can prove this to yourself. With the first goal achievement, you are on your way! You experience an inner feeling of knowing and feeling that you have brought about a change for which you are responsible.

Breast health can be the beginning goal for a new lifestyle and a healthier, happier you! Get used to being really happy. It's going to happen!

Chapter Nineteen

Visualization and Relaxation

$\mathcal{V}$ISUALIZATION

We are visualizing every moment; it is an extremely important part of our creative nature. We create pictures of what we see, or what we believe we see, which is called perceiving. The pictures we create are our perspective—our viewpoint. Our perspective is affected by our background, our education, our beliefs, our biases, our experiences, and our expectations. Ask any two people, who see an incident, to describe it and compare their stories. Each description will have been affected by their perspectives.

We can consciously use visualization to create health, attain goals, and change lifestyle. Remember, "As a man [woman] thinketh, so he [she] is!" Every thought carries a picture, whether we consciously see it or not. If we have had habits of thinking, feeling, and talking negatively, we can begin to make a conscious effort to "see" ourselves, others, and the world through "new eyes," a

new perspective. A Relaxation and Visualization Guide
has been included to assist you (see page 155).

RELAXATION

Relaxation is the balance for activity and exercise,
and is equally important. Taking time to "smell the
roses," to do loving things for ourselves and others, and
planning time to consciously relax are important plans to
incorporate into a healthier, happier *you!*

*Mankind seems to crave proof from others in
their search for truth. Any proof given outside of
yourself is but temporary—but each truth which is
proven by your own choice and conscious application
becomes truth for you.*

–Iris Ann Michael

RELAXATION AND VISUALIZATION GUIDE

Goal: To gain conscious control over your body.

Preparation:

1. Decide on a time you can practice and schedule that time, just as you would an appointment with an important person—you.

2. Select a place where you can practice—undisturbed. (Bedroom—on the bed, living room—on the sofa, or in a comfortable chair.)

3. Get comfortable. The room should be well ventilated, well lighted, and at a comfortable temperature. Remove shoes, socks, watch, glasses, or anything that would be distracting. Use a small pillow under the head and/or knees if it is more comfortable.

4. This is a learning process, and you need to remain alert and aware. If you drift off to sleep the first few times you use this guide, forgive yourself. The goal is to remain alert!

5. Sit in your chair or lie on your back, get comfortable and close your eyes. Put your arms at your side or in your lap, with the

palms of your hands turned up, allowing
the fingers to curl in a natural position.

6.   Allow and be aware that the chair or bed
     is completely supporting your body.

7.   You are going to visualize Light. Acknowl-
     edge that this comes from God.

8.   Take a few balanced breaths. Consciously
     relax.

9.   Focus your attention on your toes. Spread
     the toes apart and then let them come
     back into their natural position. As you
     visualize Light filling your toes, say si-
     lently to yourself, "My toes feel warm, re-
     laxed, and I am at PEACE."

10. Focus your attention on your feet. Con-
     sciously relax the muscles in your
     feet—pay particular attention to the
     muscles on the bottom of your feet and
     around the ankles. Visualize the Light
     filling your feet and ankles and say silent-
     ly, "My feet feel warm, relaxed, and I am
     at PEACE."

11. Focus your attention on your lower legs
     (from the ankles to the knees) and con-
     sciously relax these muscles. Visualize
     Light filling your feet and lower legs and
     say silently, "My feet and legs feel warm,
     relaxed, and I am at PEACE."

12. Focus your attention on your knees—pay
     attention to the muscles around the knees
     and in back of the knees. Visualize Light
     coming up and filling the knees and say

silently, "My knees are relaxed, comfortable, and I am at PEACE."

13. Focus your attention on your upper legs and hips and consciously relax these muscles. Visualize Light expanding to fill the upper legs and hips and say silently, "My legs feel warm, heavy, relaxed, and I am at PEACE."

14. Be aware of how you feel. This allows the memory of this controlled, relaxed "feeling" to be stored in your memory.

15. Focus your attention on the muscles of the lower back and across the front of the lower abdomen. Consciously relax these muscles. As you consciously do this, it allows the internal organs to function in a more balanced way. Visualize the Light expanding to fill the lower back muscles and the muscles covering the abdomen. Now visualize Light filling the entire abdomen—up to the diaphragm (just below the heart.) Say silently, "My lower back and abdominal muscles are relaxed and comfortable. The organs of my abdomen are filled with Light and function in a harmonious way. I am relaxed and comfortable. I am in control—and I am at PEACE."

16. Focus your attention on the muscles of your upper back and muscles covering the front of your chest. Be aware that there are muscles between each rib. Consciously relax all of these muscles. Visualize Light filling these muscles in the back and in

the front of the chest. Now expand the
Light to fill the entire chest cavity. Visualize the Light becoming more intense in the
lungs. Now "see" the Light intensifying in
the heart area. Expand the Light to fill
the *breasts* with brilliant white Light.
Hold that picture as long as you are comfortable. If the white Light changes to a
color—observe the color and watch what
happens. *Expand the Light to fill the area
under your arms. Say silently, "My
muscles are relaxed; I am in control; and I
am at PEACE."* Become aware of how you
"feel" for several moments, allowing the
memory to be clearly recorded. Say silently, "I am at PEACE. Every cell, organ and
system in my body is functioning in balance and harmony, and I am at PEACE."

17. Focus your attention on the muscles of
    your shoulders and those extending up the
    back and either side of your neck. Con-
    sciously relax these muscles and expand
    the Light to fill this entire area. Say si-
    lently, "The muscles of my shoulders and
    neck are relaxed. I am quiet, comfortable,
    and I am at PEACE."

18. Focus your attention down to your fingers
    and hands. Consciously relax these
    muscles. Become aware of how the hands
    feel warmer and more relaxed in response
    to the conscious relaxation of the rest of
    the body. Visualize the Light expanding to
    fill your fingers and hands and say silent-
    ly, "My fingers and hands are relaxed,
    warm, comfortable, and I am at PEACE."

19. Move your attention to your arms and consciously relax the muscles of your lower and upper arms. Visualize the Light filling the arms and say silently, "My arms are relaxed, comfortable, and I am at PEACE."

20. Place your attention on your face, focusing first on the large jaw muscles. With your mouth closed, allow the jaws to open in a relaxed position. See the Light filling these muscles. Pay special attention to the "hinge" area of the jaw where tightness may have developed. Say silently, "My jaws are relaxed, comfortable, and I am at PEACE."

21. Focus your attention on the muscles controlling the movement of the eyes and those around the eyes. Lift the eyebrows and allow them to come back into a relaxed, comfortable position. Visualize Light coming into and filling the eyes and see Light coming from the center of the brain, pouring out through the eyes. Say silently, "My eyes are relaxed, comfortable, balanced, and I am at PEACE."

22. Move your attention to your forehead. Consciously lift these muscles (in a stretching motion) and then allow them to come back into a relaxed position. Visualize Light filling the forehead in a fan shape. Say silently, "My forehead is relaxed, filled with Light, and I am at PEACE. I am relaxed, I am in control, and I am at PEACE."

23. Be aware of how you feel. Your body may feel very Light, balanced and peaceful. Allow the "feeling" to register in your memory bank. Tell yourself, "I can recall this 'feeling' anytime I choose to regain control of my energies, my thoughts, feelings, what I might have said, or when I just want to rebalance."

24. Now, expand the Light to fill your head, penetrating the brain and expanding into the spinal fluid flowing down from the base of the brain. "See" the Light flowing down the entire length of the spinal column. Visualize the Light pouring out through the nerves on either side of the spinal column and blending with the Light filling the rest of your body. "See" your body filled with Light. Be aware of this "feeling." Allow the "picture" and the "feeling" to enter your memory bank. Say silently, "I am at Peace, I am in control, I feel Light, balanced, harmonious, and I am at PEACE."

25. Enjoy your consciously controlled relaxation as long as you are comfortable.

"BE STILL AND KNOW THAT I AM, GOD."

INDEX

INDEX

INDEX

A

Abdomen, 47,112,157
Ability to learn, 91
Adenoids, 48
Aging, 22, 45, 47, 86, 99, 102, 118, 126, 134, 138
Alcohol, 31
Aluminum, 86
Anaerobic, 46, 82
Ankles, 99, 156
Antenna, 73
Antibodies, 16, 33
Appendicitis, 36
Appendix, 36, 44, 45, 47
Appetite, 49, 87, 88
Arterioles, 36
Atypical cells, 46, 47
Autogenic phrase, 76, 77
Axilla, 29, 55, 57, 72
Axillary area nodes, 29

B

B-cells, 33
Baby carriers, 74
Backpacks, 31
Bacteria, 34, 45, 46, 82
Balloons, 54, 64
Beauty, 16, 67
Blood, 25, 30, 36, 39, 46, 47, 48, 55, 61, 70, 73, 74, 83, 91, 97, 98, 133
Blood acidity, 83

Blues, 118
Body chemistry, 121, 138
Body-symphony, 148
Body-temple, 16, 19, 21, 22, 30, 33, 39, 40, 43, 49, 65, 67, 99, 117, 118, 127, 138
Bowel movements, 50
Bras, 31, 73, 99
Breast bone, 48, 59, 72
Breast cancer, 39
Breast massage, 69, 70
Breath, 30, 49, 74, 75, 76, 77, 100, 112, 156
Breath holding, 75
Breathing, 30, 74, 75, 76, 77

C

Caffeine, 15, 31, 82
Cancer, 17, 39, 82, 133
Carbohydrates, 81, 82, 83
Cecum, 47
Cell metabolism, 75, 82, 91, 92, 138
Cellulite, 37, 97
Cerebral-spinal fluid, 75
Circulation, 16, 25, 54, 55, 70, 73, 74, 97, 98, 100, 101, 107, 112, 138
Circulatory system, 30, 45, 46, 61, 73
Coffee, 82, 84

163

M

N